Acknowledgement

Writing about Ebola virus is not a very easy task. Because lots of information of this epidemic virus isn't reveled at this moment. Research works are going on to discover the appropriate treatment and vaccine for this virus disease. In this book I have tried hard to show the general concept of Ebola Virus Disease (EVD). I have faced great challenges to research and analyze the effect of Ebola Virus Disease (EVD) on human body. But I have tried my best to gather all necessary information about Ebola Virus Disease (EVD) in this book.

The book is going to include the following aspects, namely introduction of the Ebola virus itself, the history of Ebola virus, the causes and symptoms of the disease, the diagnosis, the occurrence, the treatment and the preventative methods etc. The book is also going to include statistics, complications of the Ebola virus, the death rate of the disease, and the experimentations which were performed in order to identify the virus and vaccine development process of this virus.

I want to thank my family and friends who are really support me lot by providing the proper information and research materials regarding this book. Without their help I can't write this book. So I am grateful to them. I think this book will helpful for those people who wants to develop their knowledge about Ebola Virus Disease (EVD) and wants get rid of this virus disease. I hope this book will helpful for human civilization of the world.

Abstract

Ebola is an epidemic virus. This virus is very dangerous than bird flu, SARS, NIPAH (NiV) and other type of epidemic viruses. In recent days the whole people of the universe faces great challenges to remove this Ebola virus from the earth. Researchers and scientists have problems when trying to develop subsidiary diagnostic tools to aid in diagnosis of Ebola Virus Disease in the early stages and undertaking ecological researches on Ebola virus and its probable reservoir. Additionally, the research also aims to observe areas that are suspected to ascertain the disease rates. To effectively prevent Ebola outbreaks in the future, more thorough knowledge of Ebola virus's disease (EVD) natural reservoir and its spread should be gained.

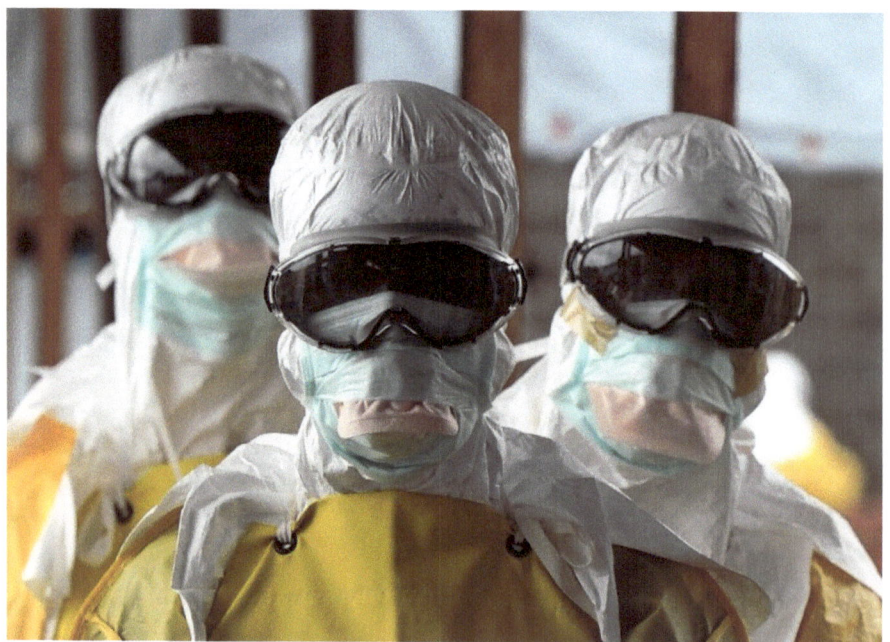

Table of Contents

1.0 Introduction

Ebola Virus Disease (EVD) is a severe disease that causes hemorrhagic fever in humans and animals. Diseases that cause hemorrhagic fevers, such as Ebola, are often fatal as they affect the body's vascular system (how blood moves through the body). This can lead to significant internal bleeding and organ failure. Ebola is a rare but deadly virus that causes bleeding inside and outside the body. As the virus spreads through the body, it damages the immune system and organs. Ultimately, it causes levels of blood-clotting cells to drop. This leads to severe, uncontrollable bleeding. The disease, also known as Ebola hemorrhagic fever or Ebola virus, kills up to 90% of people who are infected.

Ebola virus has been found in African monkeys, chimps and other nonhuman primates. A milder strain of Ebola has been discovered in monkeys and pigs in the Philippines. Marburg virus has been found in monkeys, chimps and fruit bats in Africa.

Some Key Facts about Ebola virus:

- Ebola Virus Disease (EVD), formerly known as Ebola haemorrhagic fever, is a severe, often fatal illness in humans.

- The virus is transmitted to people from wild animals and spreads in the human population through human-to-human transmission.

- The average EVD case fatality rate is around 50%. Case fatality rates have varied from 25% to 90% in past outbreaks.

- The first EVD outbreaks occurred in remote villages in Central Africa, near tropical rainforests, but the most recent outbreak in west Africa has involved major urban as well as rural areas.

- Community engagement is key to successfully controlling outbreaks. Good outbreak control relies on applying a package of interventions, namely case management, surveillance and contact tracing, a good laboratory service, safe burials and social mobilisation.

- Early supportive care with rehydration, symptomatic treatment improves survival. There is as yet no licensed treatment proven to neutralise the virus but a range of blood, immunological and drug therapies are under development.

- There are currently no licensed Ebola vaccines but 2 potential candidates are undergoing evaluation.

- Ebola is caused by infection with a virus of the family <u>Filoviridae</u>, genus Ebolavirus. There are five identified Ebola virus species, four of which are known to cause disease in humans: Ebola virus (Zaire ebolavirus); Sudan virus (Sudan ebolavirus); Taï Forest virus (Taï Forest ebolavirus, formerly Côte d'Ivoire ebolavirus); and Bundibugyo virus (Bundibugyo ebolavirus). The fifth, Reston virus (Reston ebolavirus), has caused disease in nonhuman primates, but not in humans.

- Ebola viruses are found in several African countries. Ebola was first discovered in 1976 near the Ebola River in what is now the Democratic Republic of the Congo. Since then, outbreaks have appeared sporadically in Africa.

- The natural reservoir host of Ebola virus remains unknown. However, on the basis of evidence and the nature of similar viruses, researchers believe that the virus is animal-borne and that bats are the most likely reservoir. Four of the five virus strains occur in an animal host native to Africa.

Ebola virus disease is a serious, usually fatal, disease for which there are no licensed treatments or vaccines are available at this moment. So this virus is very dangerous for whole world human civilization.

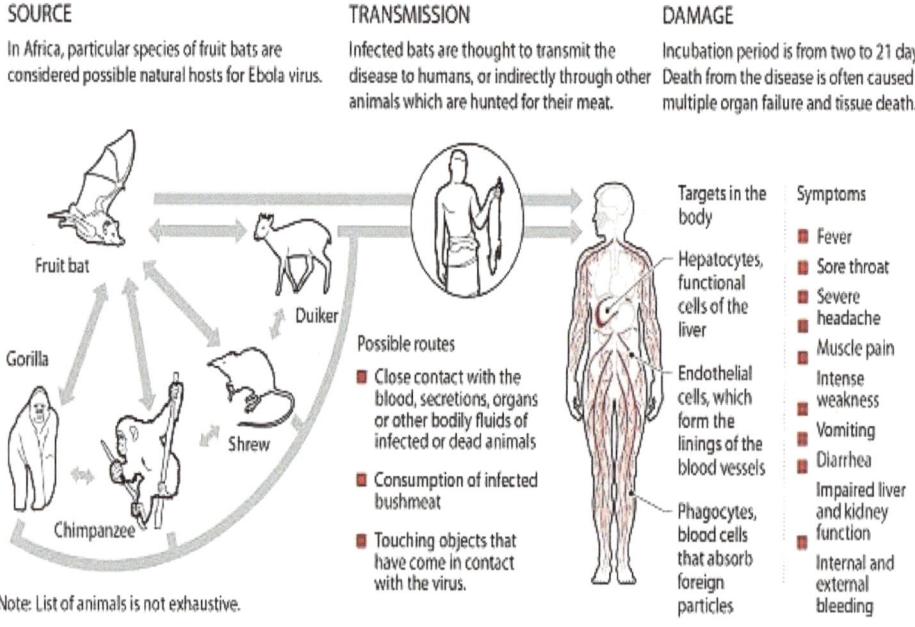

Ebola virus disease

Ebola, which first appeared in outbreaks in Sudan and DR Congo in 1976, is a severe and often fatal disease with no known specific treatment or vaccine. It has since killed more than 1,500 people in parts of Africa.

SOURCE

In Africa, particular species of fruit bats are considered possible natural hosts for Ebola virus.

TRANSMISSION

Infected bats are thought to transmit the disease to humans, or indirectly through other animals which are hunted for their meat.

DAMAGE

Incubation period is from two to 21 days. Death from the disease is often caused by multiple organ failure and tissue death.

Fruit bat

Duiker

Gorilla

Shrew

Chimpanzee

Note: List of animals is not exhaustive.

Possible routes

- Close contact with the blood, secretions, organs or other bodily fluids of infected or dead animals
- Consumption of infected bushmeat
- Touching objects that have come in contact with the virus.

Targets in the body

- Hepatocytes, functional cells of the liver
- Endothelial cells, which form the linings of the blood vessels
- Phagocytes, blood cells that absorb foreign particles

Symptoms

- Fever
- Sore throat
- Severe headache
- Muscle pain
- Intense weakness
- Vomiting
- Diarrhea
- Impaired liver and kidney function
- Internal and external bleeding

Figure 1: Ebola virus outbreak and infection process

2.0 History of Ebola Virus

In 1976, Ebola (named after the Ebola River in Zaire) first emerged in Sudan and Zaire. The first outbreak of Ebola (Ebola-Sudan) infected over 284 people, with a mortality rate of 53%. A few months later, the second Ebola virus emerged from Yambuku, Zaire, Ebola-Zaire (EBOZ). EBOZ, with the highest mortality rate of any of the Ebola viruses (88%), infected 318 people. Despite the tremendous effort of experienced and dedicated researchers, Ebola's natural reservoir was never identified.

The third strain of Ebola, Ebola Reston (EBOR), was first identified in 1989 when infected monkeys were imported into Reston, Virginia, from Mindanao in the Philippines. Fortunately, the few people who were infected with EBOR (seroconverted) never developed Ebola hemorrhagic fever (EHF). The last known strain of Ebola, Ebola Cote d'Ivoire (EBO-CI) was discovered in 1994 when a female ethologist performing a necropsy on a dead chimpanzee from the Tai Forest, Cote d'Ivoire, accidentally infected herself during the necropsy. After that incident some small Ebola outbreak occurred from 2000 to 2013 in Africa.

The most dangerous Ebola outbreak that began in March 2014 was the most serious so far. By August 13 2014 it had killed more than 5000 people across Guinea, Liberia, Ghana, Sierra Leone and Nigeria etc. The current outbreak in West Africa, (first cases notified in March 2014), is the largest and most complex Ebola outbreak since the Ebola virus was first discovered in 1976. There have been more cases and deaths in this outbreak than all others combined.

It has also spread between countries starting in Guinea then spreading across land borders to Sierra Leone and Liberia, by air (1 traveller only) to Nigeria, and by land (1 traveller) to Senegal. The most severely affected countries, Guinea, Sierra Leone and Liberia have very weak health systems, lacking human and infrastructural resources, having only recently emerged from long periods of conflict and instability. On August 8, the WHO (World Health Organization) Director-General declared this outbreak a Public Health Emergency of International Concern. A separate, unrelated Ebola outbreak began in Boende, Equateur, and an isolated part of the Democratic Republic of Congo.

. Figure 2: The outbreak of Ebola virus from 1976 to 2014

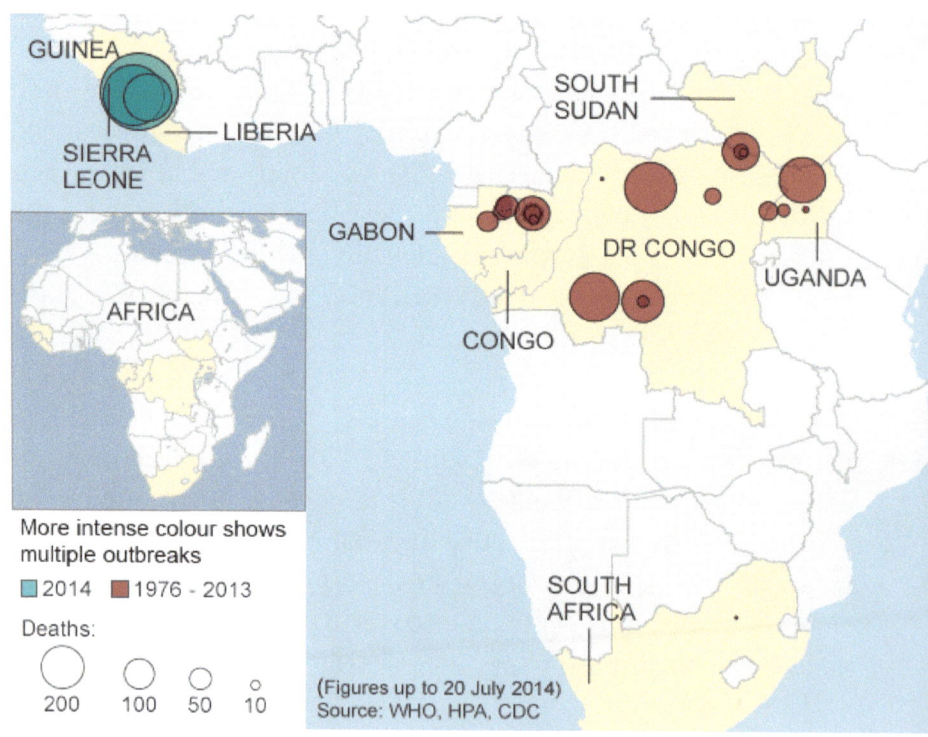

The virus family Filoviridae includes 3 genera: Cuevavirus, Marburgvirus, and Ebolavirus. There are 5 species that have been identified: Zaire, Bundibugyo, Sudan, Reston and Taï Forest. The first 3, Bundibugyo ebola virus, Zaire ebolavirus, and Sudan ebolavirus have been associated with large outbreaks in Africa. The virus causing the 2014 West African outbreak belongs to the Zaire species.

Now this outbreak also occurring in some parts of world like USA, some parts of Europe and Asia.

3.0 Causes of Ebola Virus

It is not known exactly how humans first become infected with the Ebola virus. Recent evidence suggests that humans may initially get the virus through contact with infected animals. It is thought that fruit bats of the Pteropodidae family are natural Ebola virus hosts. Ebola is introduced into the human population through close contact with the blood, secretions, organs or other bodily fluids of infected animals such as chimpanzees, gorillas, fruit bats, monkeys, forest antelope and porcupines found ill or dead or in the rainforest.

Once a person is infected, the virus can spread through person-to-person contact. Ebola then spreads through human-to-human transmission via direct contact (through broken skin or mucous membranes) with the blood, secretions, organs or other bodily fluids of infected people, and with surfaces and materials (e.g. bedding, clothing) contaminated with these fluids.

Ebola isn't as contagious as more common viruses like colds, influenza, or measles. It spreads to people by contact with the skin or bodily fluids of an infected animal, like a monkey, chimp, or fruit bat. Then it moves from person to person the same way. Those who care for a sick person or bury someone who has died from the disease often get it.

Other ways to get Ebola include touching contaminated needles or surfaces. A person can't get Ebola from air, water, or food. A person who has Ebola but has no symptoms can't spread the disease, either.

Ebola can be spread through:
- Contact with infected animals (bats, monkeys, gorillas, pigs, etc.)
- Contact with blood, body fluids or tissues of infected persons

- Contact with medical equipment, such as needles, contaminated with infected body fluids

Exposure can occur in health care Health-care workers settings when not wear appropriate protective equipment, such as masks, gowns and gloves. Health-care workers have frequently been infected while treating patients with suspected or confirmed EVD. This has occurred through close contact with patients when infection control precautions are not strictly practiced. Burial ceremonies in which mourners have direct contact with the body of the deceased person can also play a role in the transmission of Ebola.

People remain infectious as long as their blood and body fluids, including semen and breast milk, contain the virus. Men who have recovered from the disease can still transmit the virus through their semen for up to 7 weeks after recovery from illness.

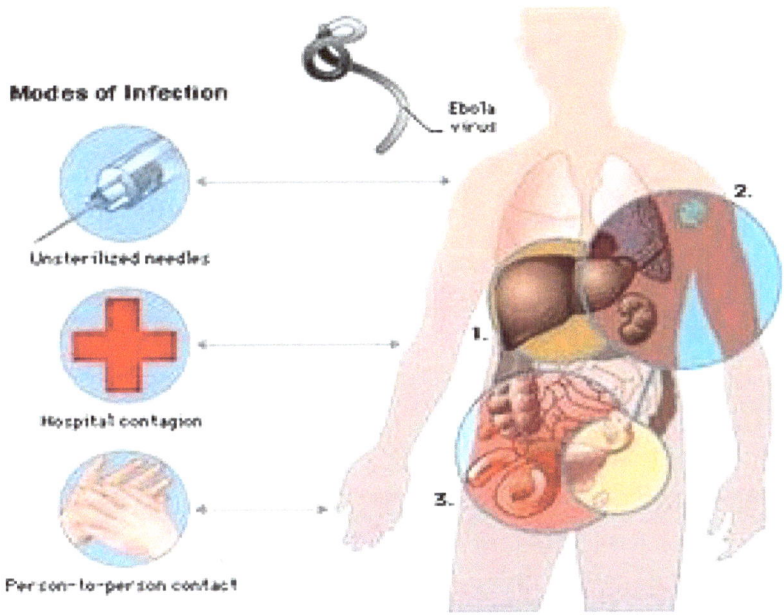

Figure 2: The causes of Ebola virus infographic image

4.0 Symptoms of Ebola Virus Infection in Human Body

The symptoms of Ebola can feel like the flu or other illnesses. As the disease gets worse, it causes bleeding inside the body, as well as from the eyes, ears, and nose. Humans are not infectious until they develop symptoms. First symptoms are the sudden onset of fever fatigue, muscle pain, headache and sore throat. Some people will vomit or cough up blood, have bloody diarrhea, and get a rash. This is followed by vomiting symptoms of impaired kidney and liver function, and in some cases, both internal and external bleeding (e.g. oozing from the gums, blood in the stools). Laboratory findings include low white blood cell and platelet counts and elevated liver enzyme

Symptoms show up 2 to 21 days after infection and usually include:

Initial symptoms include:
- Sore throat
- Fever
- Chills
- Muscle pain and weakness
- High fever
- Headache
- Joint and muscle aches
- Weakness
- Stomach pain
- Lack of appetite

Additional symptoms include:

- rash
- nausea, vomiting and diarrhea
- haemorrhaging (bleeding from inside and outside the body)

Symptoms of EVD are similar to those of other viral haemorrhagic fevers, such as Marburg, and of infectious diseases like malaria or typhoid. Diagnosis can be difficult, especially if only a single case is involved.

Some people who get infected with the Ebola virus are able to recover, although, according to the WHO (World Health Organization) and, based on previous outbreaks, up to 90% of those infected with Ebola may die.

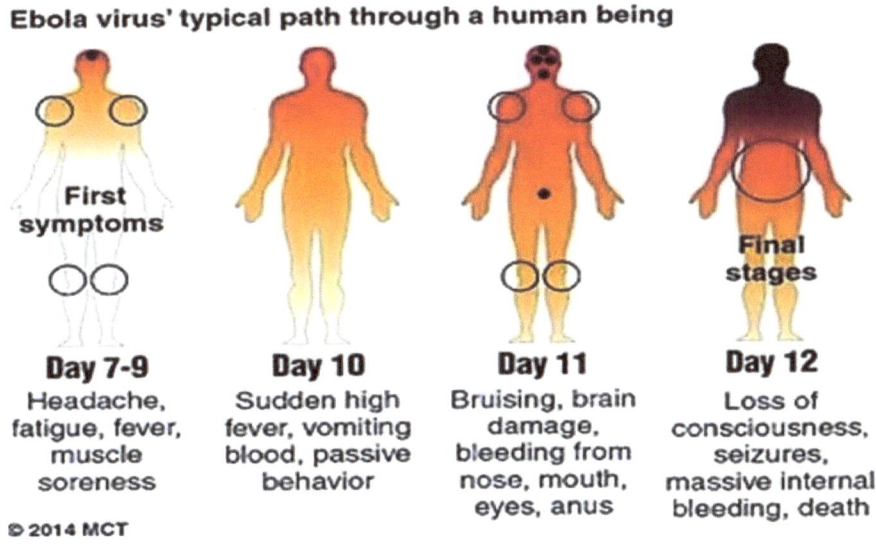

Ebola virus' typical path through a human being

First symptoms

Final stages

Day 7-9
Headache, fatigue, fever, muscle soreness

Day 10
Sudden high fever, vomiting blood, passive behavior

Day 11
Bruising, brain damage, bleeding from nose, mouth, eyes, anus

Day 12
Loss of consciousness, seizures, massive internal bleeding, death

© 2014 MCT

Figure 3: The infection process of Ebola virus in human body

What to do if a person become infected

Call a health care provider immediately if:
- You are showing some of the above symptoms **and**
- You or anyone in your household has recently travelled to an area where there is a confirmed Ebola virus outbreak.

Describe your symptoms and mention your recent travel over the phone before your appointment, so that health care staff can arrange to see you safely without potentially exposing themselves or others to the virus.

Sometimes it's hard to tell if a person has Ebola from the symptoms alone. Doctors may test to rule out other diseases like cholera or malaria. Tests of blood and tissues also can diagnose Ebola. If you have Ebola, you'll be isolated from the public immediately to prevent the spread.

5.0 Ebola Virus Disease Diagnosis Process

Ebola is diagnosed based on travel history, symptoms and laboratory testing. It can be difficult to distinguish EVD from other infectious diseases such as malaria, typhoid fever and meningitis. Confirmation that symptoms are caused by Ebola virus infection are made using the following investigations:

- Antibody-capture enzyme-linked immunosorbent assay (ELISA)
- Antigen-capture detection tests
- Serum neutralization test
- Reverse transcriptase polymerase chain reaction (RT-PCR) assay
- Electron microscopy
- Virus isolation by cell culture.
- Enzyme-linked immunosorbent assay (ELISA)
- Reverse transcriptase polymerase chain reaction (PCR)

Ebola and Marburg hemorrhagic fevers are difficult to diagnose because early signs and symptoms resemble those of other diseases, such as typhoid and malaria. If doctors suspect you have Ebola or Marburg viruses, they use blood tests to quickly identify the virus, including:

Samples from patients are an extreme biohazard risk; laboratory testing on non-inactivated samples should be conducted under maximum biological containment conditions.

6.0 Treatment and Vaccine for Ebola Virus Disease

There is currently no specific licensed treatment or vaccine for EVD. Patients are treated for their symptoms. Supportive care-rehydration with oral or intravenous fluids- and treatment of specific symptoms, improves survival. There is as yet no proven treatment available for EVD. However, a range of potential treatments including blood products, immune therapies and drug therapies are currently being evaluated. No licensed vaccines are available yet, but 2 potential vaccines are undergoing human safety testing. No antiviral medications have proved effective in treating infection with either virus. Supportive hospital care includes:

Treatment options include:

- Providing fluids

- Maintaining blood pressure

- Providing oxygen as needed

- Maintenance of oxygen status and blood pressure

- Replacing lost blood treating other infections that develop

- Replacement of lost blood and clotting factors

- Supportive care in an intensive care unit.

- Strict isolation to prevent the infection from spreading

If you develop any or all the symptoms of EVD and you have travelled to a country where there is a current Ebola outbreak, call your health care provider as soon as possible. The sooner you get treatment, the better your chances for recovery.

Both Ebola and Marburg hemorrhagic fevers lead to death for a high percentage of people who are affected. As the illness progresses, it can cause:

- Multiple organ failure
- Severe bleeding
- Jaundice
- Delirium
- Seizures
- Coma
- Shock

One reason the viruses are so deadly is that they interfere with the immune system's ability to mount a defense. But scientists don't understand why some people recover from Ebola and Marburg and others don't.

For people who survive, recovery is slow. It may take months to regain weight and strength, and the viruses remain in the body for weeks. People may experience:

- Hair loss

- Sensory changes

- Liver inflammation (hepatitis)

- Weakness

- Fatigue

- Headaches

- Eye inflammation

- Testicular inflammation

7.0 Ebola Virus Disease Prevention Plan

Prevention of a disease is better than cure. EVD Prevention Plan focuses on avoiding contact with the viruses. The following precautions can help prevent infection and spread of Ebola and Marburg.

- **Avoid areas of known outbreaks.** Before traveling to Africa, find out about current epidemics by checking the Centers for Disease Control and Prevention website.
- **Wash your hands frequently.** As with other infectious diseases, one of the most important preventive measures is frequent hand-washing. Use soap and water, or use alcohol-based hand rubs containing at least 60 percent alcohol when soap and water aren't available.
- **Avoid bush meat.** In developing countries, avoid buying or eating the wild animals, including nonhuman primates, sold in local markets.
- **Avoid contact with infected people.** In particular, caregivers should avoid contact with the person's body fluids and tissues, including blood, semen, vaginal secretions and saliva. People with Ebola or Marburg are most contagious in the later stages of the disease.
- **Follow infection-control procedures.** If you're a health care worker, wear protective clothing, such as gloves, masks, gowns and eye shields. Keep infected people isolated from others. Dispose of needles and sterilize other instruments.
- **Don't handle remains.** The bodies of people who have died of Ebola or Marburg disease are still contagious. Specially organized and trained teams should bury the remains, using appropriate safety equipment.

Other EVD prevention plan includes:

1. Avoid direct contact with blood, saliva, vomit, urine and other bodily fluids of people with EVD or unknown illnesses:

- Avoid direct contact with bodies of people who died of EVD or unknown illnesses.

- Avoid contact with any medical equipment, such as needles, contaminated with blood or bodily fluids.

- If you are a health care worker, practice strict infection control measures. This includes isolating infected individuals and properly using personal protective equipment (gowns, masks, goggles and gloves).

- If you are a health care worker, properly use and disinfect instruments and equipment used to treat or care for patients with Ebola—like needles and thermometers—before throwing them out.

2. Avoid close contact with wild animals and avoid handling wild meat:

Avoid potential carriers, both live and dead, since both can spread the virus. Potential carriers of the virus include:

- Chimpanzees

- Gorillas

- Monkeys

- Forest antelope

- Pigs

- Porcupines, and
- Fruit bats

3. Know the symptoms of EVD and see a health care provider if they develop:

- Closely monitor your health during and after travel. Seek medical attention immediately if a fever and any other symptoms arise during or after travel.

- If you develop symptoms, be sure to tell your health care provider that you have travelled to a region where EVD was present.

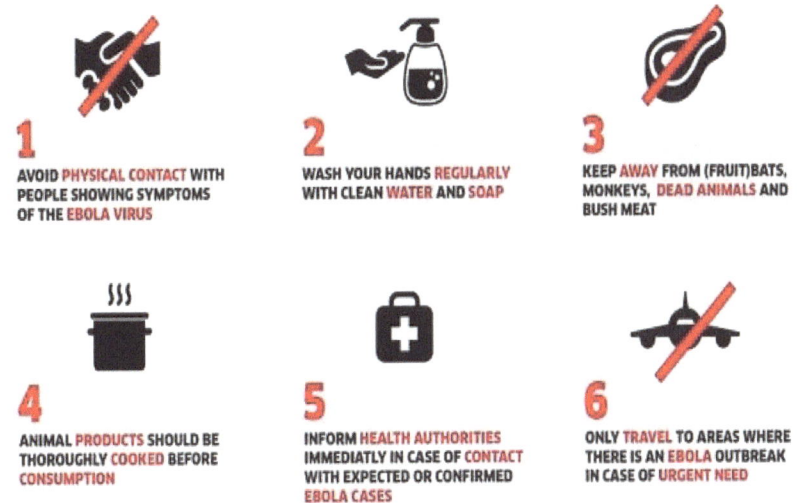

Figure 4: An infographic image of Ebola virus disease prevention plan

8.0 Controlling EVD Infection in Health-Care Settings

Health-care workers should always take standard precautions when caring for patients, regardless of their presumed diagnosis. These include basic hand hygiene, respiratory hygiene, use of personal protective equipment (to block splashes or other contact with infected materials), safe injection practices and safe burial practices.

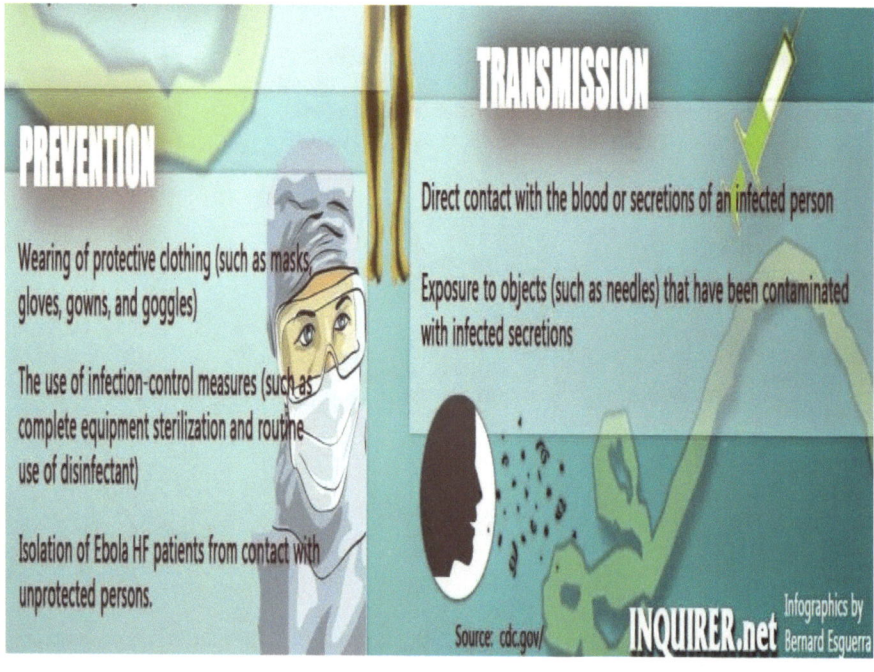

Figure 5: An infographic image of controlling EVD infection in health-care settings

Health-care workers caring for patients with suspected or confirmed Ebola virus should apply extra infection control measures to prevent contact with the patient's blood and body fluids and contaminated surfaces or materials such as clothing and bedding. When in close contact (within 1 metre) of patients with EBV, health-care workers should wear face protection (a face shield or a medical mask and goggles), a clean, non-sterile long-sleeved gown, and gloves (sterile gloves for some procedures).

Laboratory workers are also at risk. Samples taken from humans and animals for investigation of Ebola infection should be handled by trained staff and processed in suitably equipped laboratories.

9.0 Advice for EVD Health-Care Professionals

Health professionals in the different parts of the world are advised to be vigilant for the recognition, reporting and prompt investigation of patients with symptoms of Ebola virus disease (EVD) and other similar diseases that can cause viral hemorrhagic fevers.

Person-to-person transmission of Ebola virus is primarily associated with direct contact with blood and body fluids. Healthcare workers caring for patients with suspected or confirmed EVD should apply strict infection control precautions.

Pathogen Safety Data: Health professionals must maintain pathogen safety data of EVD infected person.

Case Identification: Health professionals should follow WHO (World Health Organization) EVD case identification plan.

Reporting: Patients under investigation for EVD should be reported immediately to local public health authorities as per jurisdictional protocols in the respective province or territory of a country.

Ebola Specimen Testing: Laboratories receiving specimens from patients under investigation for EVD must be aware that improper handling of these specimens poses serious risk to the health of laboratory personnel. Consult the WHO (World Health Organization) interim biosafety guidelines for laboratories handling specimens from patients under investigation for Ebola virus disease before any testing occurs. The decision for specimen collection and testing should be predicated on the clinical status of the patient and based on an on-going risk assessment.

Clinical Care: Clinical symptoms of Ebola include severe acute viral illness consisting of sudden onset of fever, malaise, myalgia, severe headache, conjunctival injection, pharyngitis, vomiting, diarrhea that can be bloody, and impaired kidney and liver function. It is often accompanied by a maculopapular or petechial rash that may progress to purpura. Bleeding from gums, nose, injection sites and gastrointestinal tract occurs in about 50% of patients. Dehydration and significant wasting occur as the disease progresses.

In severe cases, the hemorrhagic diathesis may be accompanied by leucopenia; thrombocytopenia; hepatic, renal and central nervous system involvement; or shock with multi-organ dysfunction.

Treatment: There is currently no licensed treatment or vaccine for EVD. Treatment is supportive, and is directed at maintaining renal function and electrolyte balance, and at combating hemorrhage and shock.

Health care workers can prevent infection by wearing masks, gloves, and goggles whenever they come into contact with people who may have Ebola virus disease.

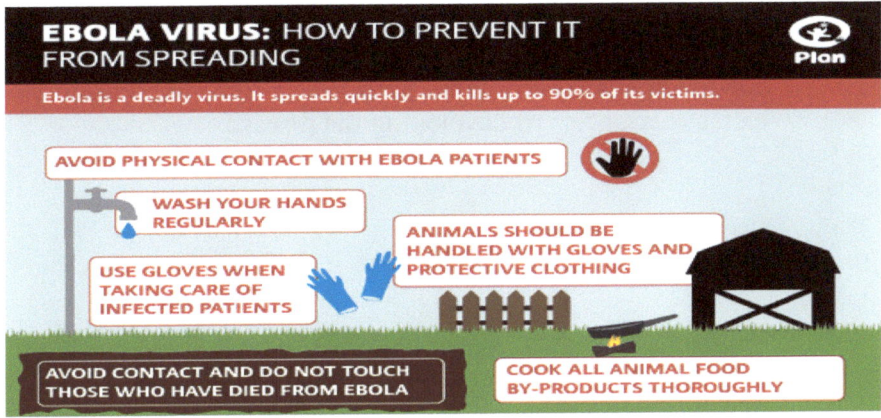

Figure 6: An infographic image for EVD health professionals

10.0 Risk Factors of Ebola Virus Disease

For most people, the risk of getting Ebola or Marburg viruses (hemorrhagic fevers) is low. The best way to avoid catching the disease is by not traveling to areas where the virus is found. The risk increases if you:

- **Travel to Africa.** You're at increased risk if you visit or work in areas where Ebola virus or Marburg virus outbreaks have occurred.

- **Conduct Animal Research.** People are more likely to contract the Ebola or Marburg virus if they conduct animal research with monkeys imported from Africa or the Philippines.

- **Provide Medical or Personal Care.** Family members are often infected as they care for sick relatives. Medical personnel also can be infected if they don't use protective gear, such as surgical masks and gloves.

- **Prepare People for Burial.** The bodies of people who have died of Ebola or Marburg hemorrhagic fever are still contagious. Helping prepare these bodies for burial can increase your risk of developing the disease.

11.0 Ebola Vaccine Development Efforts

Currently, there is no FDA-approved Ebola vaccine available to individuals; consequently, there is two Ebola vaccine that the FDA or the CDC considers "safe" as of October 2014. However, there is a lot of activity going on related to the development of a safe and effective Ebola vaccine. Consequently, the answer about an available, safe anti-Ebola vaccine may change in the near future.

For background information, readers should know that the Ebola virus is very infectious and is transmitted easily from person to person; it is a deadly viral infection that may kill 60%-90% of humans that it infects. Ebola virus infections damage blood vessels and can cause internal bleeding, shock, and eventually death. Until recently, Ebola viral infections were contained by isolating those few people infected in small settlements in several African countries.

However, in 2014, a large outbreak of Ebola infections occurred in several East African countries (Liberia, Nigeria, Sierra Leone, and Guinea) and, to date, over 5000 people have died from this infection. This is the largest Ebola outbreak ever recorded. Since there is no safe or effective vaccine and no readily available drugs that are effective in treating the disease, there is concern that this outbreak will continue and spread into many other countries.

Prevention of Ebola viruses from infecting humans is the best way to protect individuals. In general, this is done by isolating individuals who can transmit the viruses and/or by vaccinating uninfected individuals with a safe and effective vaccine. Isolating individuals who are infected is the current method used to protect uninfected people from Ebola viruses, but unfortunately, in this current outbreak, isolation techniques have not been very effective.

Vaccine development began in 2003 against Ebola viruses but none currently are available. However, because of this Ebola virus outbreak, the NIH (National Institutes of Health) of USA announced that initial treatment testing of an investigational vaccine to prevent Ebola virus disease will begin in September 2014. This phase one clinical trial will help investigators at the NIH and GlaxoSmithKline (GSK) determine the safety and efficacy of a new vaccine against Ebola. Another major trial of a vaccine will occur this fall; this vaccine is being developed by the Public Health Agency of Canada and NewLink Genetics Corp. In addition, the NIH has partnered with the British consortium to test the National Institutes of Allergy and Infectious Diseases/GSK vaccine in the United Kingdom and in the West African countries of Gambia and Mali.

Recent Ebola Vaccine Development Efforts: The World Health Organization says that efforts are on track to distribute an experimental Ebola vaccine in West Africa in January.

Two potential vaccines are now being tested for safety in people, and Russia is developing another one. While quantities will be limited, scientists say even a relatively small supply of vaccine can help bring the epidemic under control.

There's no guarantee that any vaccine will be effective, so it's good that several are in the pipeline. That includes an Ebola vaccine being developed by GlaxoSmithKline, which has already been tested in a small number of volunteers in the U.S., Europe and Africa. Marie-Paule Kieny, assistant director-general for health systems and innovation at the World Health Organization, says a Canadian vaccine licensed to NewLink Genetics in Ames, Iowa, is now being tested in people as well, at the Walter Reed National Military Medical Center and the National Institutes of Health, near Washington, D.C.

Next month, those trials will be expanded to include several hundred volunteers in Europe. Those tests will involve 250 doses of each of these two front-running vaccine candidates, "and these data are absolutely crucial to allow decision-making on what dose level should go into the testing in Africa," Kieny says.

That's a critical question at the moment, because nobody now knows whether a tiny dose or a large dose would be required to protect someone from the Ebola virus. The largest dose in these tests will be nearly 1,000 times larger than the smallest dose.

"Everybody would like to have the lowest dose because, of course, you could have so much more vaccine than if it's the highest dose," Kieny says.

Health officials are hoping to have tens of thousands of doses available starting in January. But that could present a major manufacturing challenge, especially if each shot needed to contain a huge dose of the vaccine. And while these two potential vaccines are the farthest along, they aren't alone. Three others are in earlier development stages at U.S. companies, and "some vaccines are also in development in Russia," Kieny told a WHO news conference in Geneva on Tuesday. "So we are in contact with Russians to see when they could be available for testing in Africa, and what type of doses, in terms of quantity, could be available in the months to come."She says it's not clear whether the Russian scientists have already started safety testing in people.

Until quite recently, public health officials figured that a vaccine would come along too late to be of any use in controlling the current Ebola outbreak. But that attitude is changing.
"We could use a strategy similar to the ring vaccination strategy that was used in the smallpox eradication program," says Stephen Morse, an epidemiologist at Columbia University's Mailman School of Public Health.

The concept of ring vaccination is that you wouldn't need to immunize the many millions of residents in the affected West African countries. Instead, if health officials can see where the disease is heading next, they can focus on immunizing people who will soon be in harm's way.That of course includes health care workers, who are at highest risk right now."That would not require large amounts of vaccine," Morse says, "but it probably would limit the spread of the epidemic considerably."

Using this strategy, the vaccine wouldn't have to be perfectly effective, and you wouldn't even need to vaccinate all people who are at risk in order to put brakes on the epidemic.
Drugs to treat Ebola would help as well.

Kieny says the French government plans to test a Japanese antiviral drug called Favipiravir in Guinea. And there's an international partnership coordinated by England's Oxford University to bring a half-dozen other potential drugs into the region as well.

She says the partnership is now visiting sites in the three African countries to identify which treatment centers would be adequate and would also be willing to participate in the testing of drugs. Of course, public health officials responsible for stopping Ebola are still relying most heavily on the tried-and-true method: finding people who are sick and isolating them so the disease stops spreading.

Finally, NIH is supporting two other experimental vaccine producers (Crucell and Profectus Biosciences) and is collaborating with Thomas Jefferson University to develop a vaccine based on the established rabies vaccine. NIH hopes that one or more of these experimental vaccines may be shown to be safe and effective against Ebola virus infections by late 2014 or early in 2015. Most of the companies and even the U.S. government hold patents on each type of anti-Ebola vaccine. Vaccines are designed to stimulate an immune response against Ebola viruses that will protect uninfected individuals who are exposed to live Ebola viruses. The vaccines do not contain live Ebola viruses, only antigens or parts of the virus that can stimulate a protective immune response. The vaccines cannot cause Ebola infections. WHO (World Health Organization) declares that they will produce and supply 100000 Ebola vaccines in 2015.

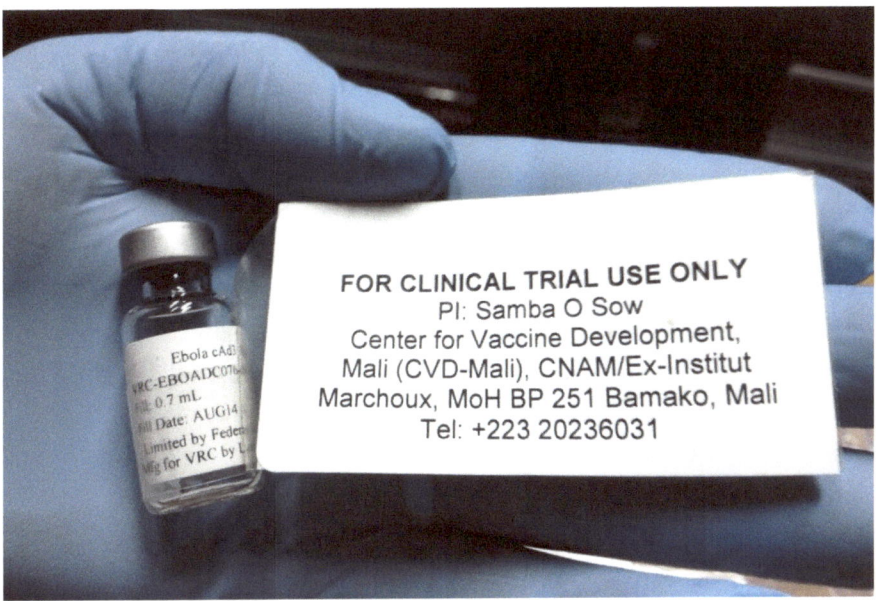

Figure 7: An image of experimental Ebola vaccine, developed by the U.S. & Canada government, is just one of several undergoing small-scale, preliminary testing.

12.0 Conclusion

Ebola virus (EBOV) is considered to be one of the most belligerent contagious agents and has an ability to cause highly fatal hemorrhagic fever syndrome that results in human and non-human primate's death (NHPs) during the days of exposure. The first notification of the virus was mentioned in the Ebola River valley in Zaire for the time of an outburst in 1976. Moreover, the outbursts have appeared in Africa over the following 27 years, with death rates that differ from 50 to 90%. In Central Africa, for the last three years outbursts have been recognized every year, the most recent of which proceeded in the Republic of the Congo with the amount of victims more than 125, according to the World Health Organization.

It has been proven that the Ebola virus can be transferred from one human being to another by means of bodily contact. The common geographic territory considered being mostly influenced by divergent subtypes of the Ebola virus is Central Africa, especially the cities of Zaire, Sudan, and Gabon.

The precise derivation, positions, and natural habitats, which are also known as natural reservoirs of Ebola virus, continue to be unidentified. Nevertheless, according to the available substantiation and the features of the same viruses, researchers claim that the virus is zoonotic (animal-borne), with 4 out of 5 subtypes that happen in animal hosts close to Africa.

The Ebola virus can be diagnosed with the particular antigens discovered in blood samples, isolation of virus in cell cultures, or identification of IgM and IgG antibodies. ELISA (Enzyme-linked immunosorbent assay) tests are frequently utilized in order to identify viruses. It should be mentioned that all tests are performed in the most rigorous laboratory conditions aiming to secure scientists and patients.

There is considered to be no identified treatment for Ebola virus disease. Therefore, contaminated patients are treated by means of utilizing antiviral drugs, including ribavirin. Another method is a generally supportive therapy which restores endovenous fluids, keeps blood pressure in a good condition, and controls other bodily functions.

The preventive methods of Ebola HF in Africa face numerous challenges. It happens, since the originality and location of the natural reservoir of Ebola virus are unexplored. Consequently, there are only few minor established initial preventive measures.

The good news is WHO (World Health Organization) and many nations of the world are trying to develop Ebola vaccine. And they have already shown some outstanding effort in this vaccine development research and analysis. So we can hope that human civilization will remove this virus from our world and develop proper treatment plan, vaccine for this Ebola virus disease.

References and Bibliography

Chepurnov, A., Bakulina, L., Dadaeva, A., Ustinova, E., & Chepurnova, T. (2009). Inactivation of Ebola virus with a surfactant nanoemulsion. *Transfusion, 49*(Suppl.), 72-74.

Dowell, S. F., Mukunu, R., Ksiazek, T. G., Khan, A. S., Rollin, P. E., Peters, C. J. and the   Commission de Lutte contreles Epidémies à Kikwit. (1999). Transmission of Ebola hemorrhagic fever: A study of risk factors in family members, Kikwit, Zaire. *The Journal of Infectious Diseases, 179* (Suppl. 1), 87-91.

Falco M. (2012). Could the Ebola outbreak spread to the U.S.? Retrieved from <http://edition.cnn.com/2012/07/31/health/the-ebola-outbreak>

International Study Team. (1978). Ebola hemorrhagic fever in Sudan, 1976. *Bulletin of the World Health Organization, 56*(2), 247-270.

Lovgren S. (2003). Where Does Ebola Hide Between Epidemics? Retrieved from <http://news.nationalgeographic.com/news/2003/02/0219_030219_e bolaorigin.html>

MacNeil A., Farnon E., Cannon D., Reed Z., Towner J., Nichol S., Ksiazek T., Rollin P. (2010).   Proportion of Deaths and Clinical Features in Bundibugyo Ebola Virus   Infection,   Uganda. Retrieved   from   http://wwwnc.cdc.gov/eid/article/16/12/10-0627_article.htm

Olival K., Islam A., Anthony S., Epstein H., Daszak P. (2013). Ebola Virus Antibodies in Fruit   Bats, Bangladesh. Retrieved from <http://wwwnc.cdc.gov/eid/article/19/2/12-   0524_article.htm>

Report of an International Commission. (1978). Ebola hemorrhagic fever in Zaire, 1976. *Bulletin of the World Health Organization, 56*(2), 271-293. Retrieved from <http://whqlibdoc.who.int/bulletin/1978/Vol56No2/bulletin_1978_5 6(2)_271-293.pdf>

Peters, C. (1999). An introduction to Ebola: The virus and the disease. *The Journal of Infectious*

Diseases, 179 (Suppl. 1), ix-xvi. Retrieved from <http://www.eva.mpg.de/primat/ebola_workshop/pdf/Peters_andLe DucEbola_review.pdf>

Weingartl, H., Embury-Hyatt, C., Nfon, C., Leung, A., Smith, G., & Kobinger, G. (2012).Transmission of Ebola virus from pigs to non-human primates. *Scientific Reports, 2*, 811.

About the Author

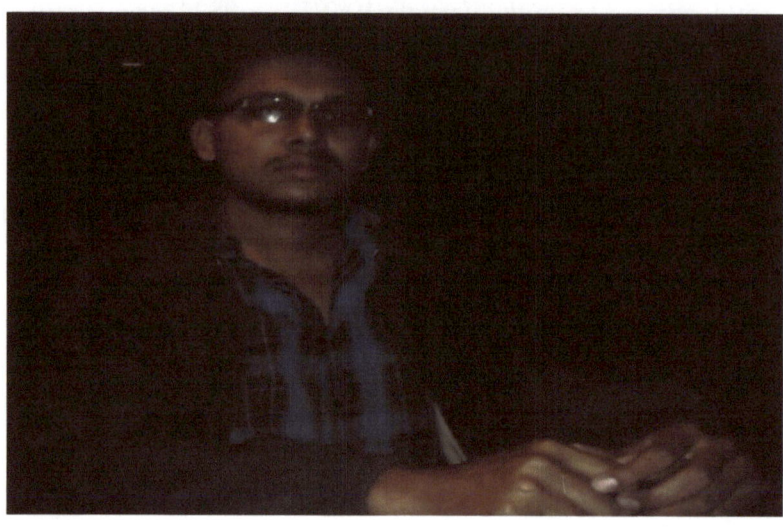

Ghazi Mokammel Hossain is a professional e-book, article, research paper, report and creative writer. He has written many articles, research papers, report and creative articles. He is also a freelance writer and researcher. The author lives in Dhaka, Bangladesh. He was born in 31 December 1993. The name of his father is Ghazi Mozammel Hossain and his mother name is Syeda Taskin Ara. He has passed his S.S.C exam from Narinda Govt. High School, Dhaka under Dhaka Board in 2008 and passed his H.S.C exam from Ideal Commerce College, Dhaka under Dhaka Board in 2010. Now he is studying in BBA (Honors) 4th year in Victoria University Bangladesh. He has also completed Computer Science and Engineering certificate course in 2011. He has published his first book called "IPv4 IP6 Technology & Implementation" in Amazon kindle and Createspace.com on 2013. He has published his second book called "Introduction to Network on Chip Routing Algorithms" on 2014. And he has also published his third book called "Fundamental of API Based Financial Engineering" on 2014. Playing football, Cricket, PC games, Reading fictional, non-fictional book, research paper, cycling and mountain climbing are his favorite hobbies.

Detail Information of the Book:

Authored by: Ghazi Mokammel Hossain

Editing and Proofread by: i. Dr. Robert Alex
ii. Dr. Taylor Brown
iii. Dr. Oliver Alan Mayer

Designed by: Ghazi Mokammel Hossain

Publications Format: Amazon Kindle E-Book format, Amazon Createspace Paper back format

Edition No: First Edition

Publication From: Dhaka, Bangladesh

Version: International Version

Published by: GM Publishers, associated with Amazon Kindle Direct Publishing & Createspace

ISBN:

ISBN-13: 978-1502978257

ISBN-10: 1502978253 (The book has been assigned a CreateSpace ISBN)

Contact Address:

Email address: gmjon21@gmail.com
Skype Id: gmhossain380
Phone no: +8801674950802